Guidelines for Basic Computer Education in Nursing

Judith S. Ronald, EdD, RN
School of Nursing
State University of New York at Buffalo

Diane J. Skiba, PhD
Graduate School of Nursing
University of Massachusetts Medical Center
Worcester, Massachusetts

Pub. No. 41-2177

National League for Nursing • New York

Manufactured in the United States of America.

Preface

Nurses have traditionally adopted and used new technology in their care of patients: for example, the thermometer, the sphygmomanometer, the cardiac monitor, and the microcomputer-based IV regulator. Each tool was readily adopted after its utility was demonstrated. As such, the new tools extended nurses' capabilities and allowed them to make observations and give care that was not possible without the technology. Importantly, many of these technological tools affected care in ways that could not have been predicted before their adoption. Some effects have been quite positive, others not as positive.

Thus nurses, as professionals, learned firsthand about the double-edged sword of technology. Nurses recognized that at the same time that the tools improved care they also imposed further demands on professional nurses as caregivers. Thus it is with technological tools: the care benefits are balanced by increased demands on users of the tools. For example, computers, as tools, contribute to the generation of data. As a result, the nurse must manage more and more data. When the increased amounts of data are analyzed, new patterns of knowledge and information become available.

It is in this context of technology and information that Drs.

Ronald and Skiba have prepared this publication on integrating computer content into nursing educational curricula. Their aim is to help nursing educators prepare students to use the computer as a tool for an information-intensive profession. For if the computer has helped create an information explosion, it also provides us with our best means of managing the data available to us. Our students must be prepared to function in the real world of technology and information; therefore, they must be able to manage the computer and make it work for them.

This book is divided into three chapters, plus extensive resources and appendices. Chapter 1 presents the idea of a computer-education continuum that serves as a framework for curriculum planning. Use of the continuum allows faculty to decide on their students' desired proficiency in computer use and adapt their curriculum planning to fit the predetermined end point.

Chapter 2 describes in detail the decision making involved in integrating computer content into the nursing curriculum. The authors take the reader through the process step by step, from the defining of learning objectives to final evaluation of the curriculum change. Chapter 3 sets out a detailed content outline of topics from which the faculty can choose in designing the computer curriculum, including descriptions of proposed learning activities to accompany each unit.

The curriculum decision-making process the authors describe is useful for both basic and continuing education programs. After clearly delineating the curriculum decisions that must be made, the authors present useful suggestions for detailed needs assessments.

Throughout this book, the range of topics considered and content suggested is comprehensive. Included is a set of up-to-date resources for faculty planning of actual course materials. In addition, the manuscript was extensively reviewed in draft form by members of the computer forum executive committee and nurses from the academic and service sectors for completeness, currency, and relevance. I commend it to your use in planning for this important curriculum component.

— *Susan Grobe, PhD, RN, FAAN*
Associate Professor
The University of Texas at Austin
Chairperson
National Forum on Computers
in Health Care and Nursing

Contents

Acknowledgments

We dedicate this manuscript to our students, whose thirst for knowledge about computers in nursing challenged us to address computer education within the curriculum.

Our sincere appreciation goes to the members of the Executive Committee of the National Forum on Computers in Health Care and Nursing for providing the initial impetus for this project: Susan Grobe, PhD, RN, FAAN, The University of Texas at Austin; William Holzemer, PhD, RN, FAAN, University of California at San Francisco; Karen A. Rieder, DNSc, RN, Office of the Assistant Secretary of Defense for Health Affairs; Roy Simpson, RN, Hospital Corporation of America; and Pat Tymchyshyn, PhD, RN, Softpat Corporation. Their encouragement, guidance, and critical review of various drafts of the manuscript contributed significantly to its development.

The assistance of the following reviewers, who read and commented on the manuscript, is also gratefully acknowledged:

The following former members of the NLN staff: Jeanine Greenfield, ScD, RN; Carl Miller, PhD, RN; and Marjory Peterson, EdD, RN.

The following additional reviewers: Jane A. Fanning, MS, RN, CNAA, Bayfront Medical Center, St. Petersburg, Florida; Carol

Hudgings, PhD, RN, Hospital Corporation of America, Nashville; Denise R. Lucas, BSN, RN, Bethesda Hospital School of Nursing, Cincinnati; Jean McClusky, MEd, RN, School of Practical Nursing, Sacred Heart Hospital, Norristown, Pennsylvania; and Mary Powell, RN, Hospital Corporation of America, Nashville. The suggestions of all of the reviewers greatly improved the content and overall organization of the monograph. However, the authors assume full responsibility for the final product.

We are grateful to the deans of our schools of nursing, Bonnie Bullough, PhD, RN, FAAN, State University of New York at Buffalo, and Kathleen Dirschel, PhD, RN, University of Massachusetts at Worcester, for their assistance and support.

In addition, we want to thank two staff members of the National League for Nursing: Franklin Schaffer, EdD, RN, deputy director, for his continuing support throughout the project; and Elaine Silverstein, editorial director, for her expert assistance.

—*Judith S. Ronald*
—*Diane J. Skiba*

1

A Framework for
Computer Education

INTRODUCTION

Learning about computers and their use presents a challenge for
all nurses and is becoming increasingly important as the use of
computer technology in nursing and health care expands, and the
nurse's role expands concomitantly to encompass the application
of this technology to patient care. If the computer is to meet the
needs of nurses as well as of health care consumers, it is crucial
that nurses be more than passive users of computer systems
developed by others. Nurses must participate actively in developing and designing computer applications in nursing service and
education as well as communicate effectively with computer and
information scientists and critically evaluate existing health
information systems.

This active involvement requires knowledge of computers and
information technology. As a consequence, educators are faced
with the problem of how to prepare nurses to meet the challenges
imposed by computers. Nursing educators are being asked to
make decisions about the specific computer knowledge and skills
that nurses need, and about where and how in the educational

1

program they should be provided. Since no universally accepted computer curriculum for nurses has been developed, this can be problematic for educators who have limited background and experience with computers. Many nursing educators do not know how to start integrating computers into the curriculum (Gothler, 1985).

Purpose

The purpose of this publication is to provide assistance to educators who are in the process of integrating computer concepts into their curricula. The guidelines presented are not a definitive statement of what nurses need to know, but rather a broad framework from which educators can develop objectives, select content, design learning activities, and choose resources. The guidelines are meant to be flexible and can be adapted by faculty to meet the computer-related needs of learners within a specific setting. It is anticipated that nursing educators will modify the guidelines to fit their specific settings. Although the guidelines have been developed primarily with school of nursing faculty in mind, many of the issues discussed are equally relevant for staff development educators in health care institutions.

The material in this document has been gathered from the literature and personal communication with educators actively involved in teaching nurses about computers and their uses in nursing. It is the authors' intention to answer some of the most frequently asked questions about the content and method for teaching nurses about computers, as well as to address important issues regarding integration of computer concepts into the nursing curriculum.

In order to achieve these goals, the authors have conceptualized these guidelines within a general curriculum development model (Torres & Stanton, 1982). First, the reader is introduced to a framework for computer education. This is followed, in the second chapter, by a graphic representation (flowchart) of the steps involved in the curriculum decision-making process and a discussion of these steps. The purpose of the flowchart and the subsequent discussion is to help faculty make decisions in the traditional areas of development of learning objectives, selection of content, identification of learning activities, placement of content, and selection of teaching and evaluation methods. Given the breadth of content related to computers, the third chapter provides a detailed outline of possible computer topics to integrate into nursing education. In addition, selected resources are included in the appendices.

FRAMEWORK

To provide a flexible and adaptable set of guidelines, the authors list here the assumptions that serve as the basis for the development of a computer education framework:

- Nurses need knowledge of computers.
- Nurses must be proactive in the use of computer technology in nursing.
- Computer education consists of both cognitive and interactive components.
- Computer education in nursing includes computer basics as well as nursing applications.
- Computer education exists along a continuum of learning experiences.
- Computer education for nurses should stress the use of the computer as a problem-solving tool.
- Nursing educators should determine the appropriate curriculum plan for their learners.
- The nurse's role with computers will expand with the increasing use of computers in health care.

Based on these assumptions, the authors developed a computer education framework consisting of a continuum of learning experiences with both cognitive and interactive components. (Fig. 1-1) **Cognitive learning** includes specific content related to basic computer concepts and applications in nursing that nurses need to function effectively in the health care delivery system. The **interactive component** refers to the skills necessary for the operation of the computer as well as the ability to use the computer as a problem-solving tool. The framework incorporates a continuum that ranges from informed user to developer. As one moves along the continuum, there is a concomitant enlargement

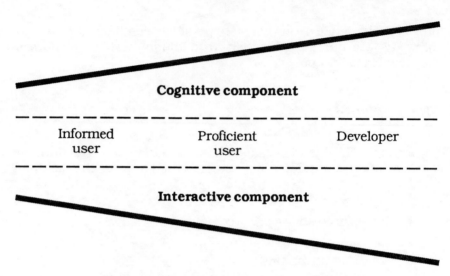

Figure 1–1. Computer education continuum.

of both the cognitive and interactive components. The authors believe that all nurses should be at the "informed user" level and that most professional nurses should reach the "proficient user" level. Only those nurses with advanced preparation will become "developers," as shown at the endpoint of the continuum.

Table 1-1 describes the expectations of learners related to the major content areas at these three points on the continuum. Necessary elements are included for both the cognitive and interactive components: for the cognitive component, basic computer concepts and applications in nursing; for the interactive component, hands-on experience with computer systems. In order to clarify the differences in learner behaviors for the points on the continuum described in Table 1-1, examples of specific learning objectives are given below:

- **Computer concepts (e.g., software)**

  Informed user: define the term "software."

  Proficient user: examine the logic behind programming.

  Developer: write an original computer program.

- **Applications (e.g., clinical practice)**

  Informed user: describe the use of the computer to generate nursing care plans.

Table 1–1. Learner expectations at three points on the basic computer education continuum.

Points on continuum	Cognitive components		Interactive components
	Basic concepts	Applications	
Informed user	Be familiar with computer terminology	Identify common applications in nursing	Operate a computer system
Proficient user	Understand basic computer concepts	Assess the relative value of existing computer systems and communicate nursing needs for the development of future systems	Use the computer as a tool to solve nursing problems
Developer	Have in-depth knowledge of computer concepts and information management	Apply systems analysis and design concepts to the development of computer applications for nursing	Use programming skills to maximize the potential of software to solve nursing problems

Proficient user: assess various approaches to computerized nursing care planning.

Developer: analyze nursing information needs to design and develop a computerized care planning system.

- **Computer interaction**

Informed user: use the computer to generate a nursing care plan.

Proficient user: manipulate information from the computerized nursing care planning system to analyze the relationship between nursing actions and patient outcomes.

Developer: develop a computerized nursing care planning system to meet the needs of a specific institution.

The cognitive and interactive objectives described above show how learners are expected to develop knowledge and skill of progressively greater depth and breadth as they move along on the continuum.

A Scenario

In order to clarify further the differences in the three points on the continuum, a scenario is presented that describes the behavior of three nurses who work in a hospital with a computerized information system and are at different points on the computer education continuum. Nurse A represents the informed user; Nurse B, the proficient user; Nurse C, the developer.

As the scene opens, Nurse A, a primary nurse on a surgical unit, is sitting at the computer terminal completing the charting. Nurse A mentions to Nurse B that there have been several patients with wound infections recently and then goes on to say:

Nurse A: I would really like to know the incidence of infections for all of the patients who have been on this unit within the last couple of weeks, as well as the organisms responsible for the infections. It seems as if this is something that the computer ought to be able to do. Is there any software available to do this?

Nurse B: Your question shows how we can use the computer as a tool to solve a nursing problem. Our hospital information system has a database management system that lets us ask for any combination of information stored on the patient's record.

Nurse A: I understand the concept of a database, but how does a database management system work?

Nurse B: A database management system is software that allows you to store comprehensive patient information in a central location and then access, manipulate, and report this information in a variety of ways.

Nurse A: How do you manipulate information to get what you want?

Nurse B: You have to use a special set of commands called a query language. The commands use Boolean operators and are easy to use.

Nurse A: Yes, I remember. Boolean operators are "and," "or," and "not," aren't they? I used them when I did a MEDLINE search in school.

Nurse B: That's right. Let's sit down at the terminal and I'll show you how quickly and easily you can get an answer to your question using the query language from our database.

Later, as the two nurses are reviewing the information they have retrieved from the database, Nurse A asks Nurse B another question:

Nurse A: Is it possible to get the same information for the whole hospital? Could we relate it to DRGs? or to other factors? Could we get a report every week, or whenever we want it?

Nurse B: I think so. Let's go talk to Nurse C.

The scene changes to Nurse C's office.

Nurse B: We're interested in conducting a study of wound infection across hospital units within DRG categories. We'd also like to look at some other factors that might be significant.

Nurse A: How can we use the database management system to do this?

Nurse C: This would be a good application for our database management system. However, I need to know exactly what you want and what data elements you are referring to.

Nurse A: What's a data element?

Nurse C: Data elements refer to specific pieces of patient information stored in the database. For example, do you want admitting DRG or discharge DRG? Specifically what other factors are you interested in?

Nurse A: I'm not sure. It sounds as if I will have to think more about what I want to know.

Nurse C: Yes you will. The other thing that I'll have to know is exactly what kind of report you need. If it doesn't fit the standard database report form, I'll have to write a special program in database language to give you what you need.

Nurse B: We'll define exactly what information we need from the database and come back to see you next week.

Nurse C: That will be fine. It would be helpful if you could also sketch out the format of the report that you would like.

2

The Curriculum Decision-Making Process

Given the framework in Chapter 1, faculty will make several decisions about integrating computers into the curriculum. This chapter will guide the faculty through the curriculum planning process with specific reference to computer technology. A flowchart is used to depict the decision-making process (Fig. 2–1). For the sake of simplicity, an essentially linear model is used. However, the authors recognize that curriculum planning occurs in a nonlinear progression with several feedback loops.

REQUIRED OR ELECTIVE?

At the beginning point on the flowchart, it is assumed that a decision has been made to incorporate computer content into the curriculum. The next critical decision made by the faculty is whether the content about computers in nursing should be required. In order to answer this question in an intelligent manner, faculty need to consider several areas: (1) fit with overall curriculum goals, (2) current educational trends, and (3) changing requirements of the health care delivery system. This is not an easy decision, but it is a critical point in the process. If the content is to

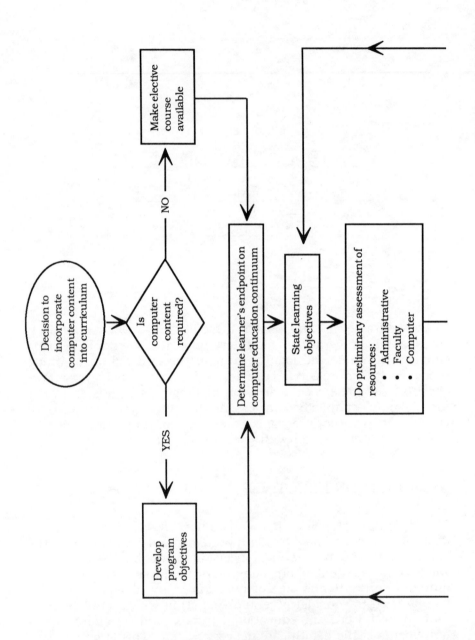

Figure 2–1. Flowchart for curriculum decision making.

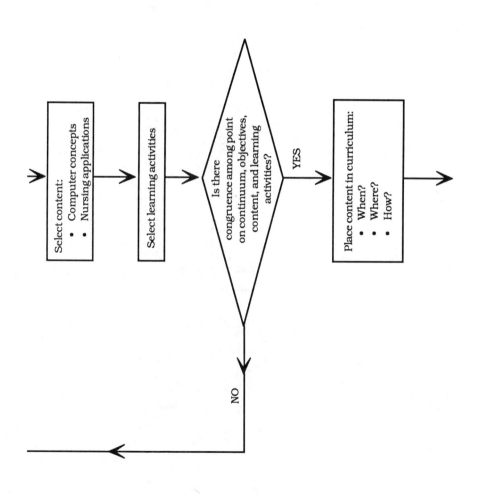

Figure 2-1. *(continued)*

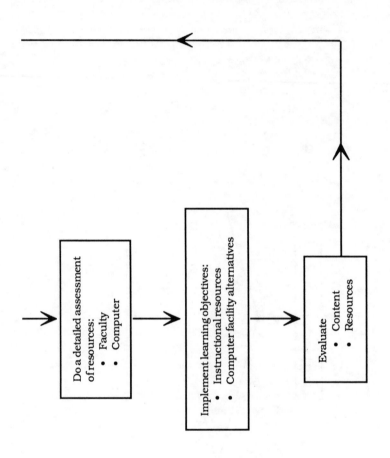

Figure 2-1. *(continued)*

be required, the faculty will either write a terminal program objective or incorporate the content into one of the existing terminal objectives. If the faculty consensus is that the content is important but should not be required for graduation, the content can be made available to students on an elective basis. Offering the content in this way implies that a program objective is not necessary.

Learners' Endpoint on Framework

As noted in the flowchart, the next step is the exploration and analysis of the computer education framework (see Chapter 1) to determine the most appropriate endpoint on the continuum for the learners (informed user, proficient user, or developer). This decision should be made by the faculty or the appropriate group (e.g., the curriculum committee) within the organization.

LEARNING OBJECTIVES

After determining the desired endpoint on the continuum, the faculty writes learning objectives that incorporate elements from both the cognitive and interactive components of the computer education framework (see Table 1-1). It is important to remember that the cognitive component includes two areas: computer concepts and applications in nursing. Thus objectives should be written for each of the three areas. Sample objectives can be found in Chapter 1.

PRELIMINARY ASSESSMENT OF RESOURCES

A preliminary assessment of resources is necessary at this point to determine the feasibility of continuing the planning process. The assessment includes examination of administrative and faculty support as well as availability of computer resources. By means of informal mechanisms, the faculty can gain insight into support for the change process and identify potential problem areas. The preliminary assessment does not eliminate the need for a more detailed assessment of faculty and computer resources, which will occur before the implementation phase.

Support from the administrator of the school of nursing is a key ingredient for the successful implementation of computer education. According to Masland (1984), the administrator's characteristics may influence the success of any computer education initiatives. During the preliminary assessment of resources, it is essential to determine your administrator's level and type of support. Level of support can range from active support to discouraging all computing efforts. The level of administrative support will depend upon three factors: knowledge of computer technology, attitude toward computer technology and information systems in health care, and experience with computer technology. Another factor that may affect administrative support is competing needs within the institution. For example, a school may be suffering from declining enrollments and faculty unrest, so the dean may decide that the introduction of computer education into the curriculum would be inappropriate at the current time.

The importance of these factors and their relationship to administrative support can not be overestimated. In a study of academic deans and computer usage, Johnson (1984) found that deans, in general, had limited knowledge of computer capabilities and did not personally use computers for managerial tasks. Walker's (1986) study concurred with these findings and concluded that "there was a general lack of planning for adoption and use of computers in the nursing educational environment."

Administrative support. In addition to level of support, the type of support your administrator provides should also be assessed. Type of support for computer efforts may include money for acquisition of faculty, hardware, and software; faculty release time for curriculum development; time for faculty development; or access to necessary resources. Administrative support can be provided within the school as well as outside the school. According to Felton and Brown (1985), "the nursing dean will need to influence policy decisions, bargain with central administrators for collegiate initiatives and disseminate and interpret information about impending decisions and new developments" (p. 7).

Given the importance of administrative support, a faculty group considering computer education initiatives should approach their administrator at the onset. Try to determine your administrator's potential level and type of support. What follows is a description of three typical administrative support scenarios.

Active administrators encourage and support computer initiatives. They may provide necessary resources (money, release time) and promote the school's efforts to central administration. These administrators usually are knowledgeable about computer technology, recognize the impact of technology and information systems on the health care system, have had experience with use of computers as productivity tools for management or administrative tasks or functions, value technology within society and health care, and have a positive attitude toward computer technology within the nursing profession.

A second type of administrator encourages the faculty to work on computer education initiatives but takes a less active stance (Masland, 1984). These administrators realize the benefits of computing in health care and nursing but are often less knowledgeable about technology and have had limited experience with use of computers as problem-solving tools. Although these administrators' knowledge and experience level is low, their attitudes are positive, so they encourage faculty to pursue the development of computer education for students. The administrator tries to provide necessary resources and will usually let the faculty take the leadership role. In some ways, this type of administrator provides philosophic support and encouragement for computer education.

The final type of administrator may actively discourage computer education initiatives. Numerous reasons can be projected to explain an administrator's lack of support for computer education. One may be the administrator's belief that other institutional needs are more important than the need for computer education (Masland, 1984). The administrator may think that the high schools or the liberal arts component of undergraduate education should be responsible for providing computer education, or that the integration of computer education within the curriculum is inconsistent with the mission and goals of the school of nursing. Another reason for lack of support could be the administrator's ignorance of computer technology and its use in nursing and inexperience with the use of the computer as a productivity tool. The administrator's negative attitude toward technology and computer applications in nursing and health care may also be a reason for the lack of support for computer education.

Faculty support. As with any change in the curriculum, it is important to determine faculty support. The faculty must be

aware of curriculum issues that may arise when computer technology is integrated into an already overloaded curriculum.
Although they value the importance of computer technology in
nursing education, priorities may have to be reexamined and
compromises made to adapt the curriculum for this change.

Computer resources. Availability of computer resources for
educational purposes, in both the school and the community,
should also be explored at this time. The number, type, and location of available computers will greatly affect both the content
and instructional methods selected for the course.

Felton (1984) has suggested a variety of questions that should be
posed when planning for computers in educational settings. The
first three sections of her checklist (preliminary planning, support, and funding and acquisition) are presented in Figure 2–2.

CONTENT

After the preliminary assessment of resources, the faculty selects
specific content to meet the learning objectives. The computer
education framework provides direction for the selection of content related to both computer concepts and applications in
nursing. Further, it indicates that those areas should have both a
cognitive and interactive component.

To help select appropriate content, an extensive topic outline of
computer content areas is provided in Chapter 3. The outline is
divided into six major sections: (1) historical perspectives, (2) basic computer concepts (e.g., information processing, hardware,
data representation, software), (3) systems analysis and design,
(4) application of the computer to nursing (clinical, administrative, educational, research), (5) the role of the nurse, and (6) professional issues related to the use of the computer in health care.
Within each major heading are detailed listings of pertinent
topics. The last two sections, which are related to roles and issues,
have been separated out in the outline, but they are integral parts
of the application content and are usually taught concurrently
with it.

This outline is intended to be used as a guide by educators in
their selection of content. It is not an exhaustive list of all
possible content, nor is it meant to imply that all content listed
must be covered in the curriculum. The faculty should modify it to

Figure 2–2. Felton's checklist for computer planning (Part I).

I. **Preliminary planning:**

   A. How does computer equipment relate to department goals or to a master plan?

   B. What is the *value* of the computer function to nursing in your department?

   C. What possibilities exist in your department or section?

     1. Instruction _____

     2. Research _____

     3. Administration _____

   D. Describe the instructional, research, or administrative use in as *much detail* as possible.

   E. How will computer activity accomplish something more efficiently or effectively?

II. **Developing support for the plan:**

   A. What support groups are available for consultation (other departments, computer stores, user groups)?

   B. Who within the department already knows how to work with computers?

   C. How many may need or want to use it?

   D. How will department, level, and/or course objectives be modified to include computer activity?

   E. Who will have the knowledge and time to provide inservice for department members and/or students?

III. **Funding and acquisition:**

   A. What are possible sources of funds and/or equipment?

   B. What is the nature of the proposal grant or request?

   C. Who could help with the proposal via previous experience with and/or proximity to the process?

Figure 2-2. *(continued)*

D. After submission of a proposal, what is the length of the funding process?
E. Have you explored alternate sources?
F. How is money allocated after the grant or proposal is approved?
G. Who monitors expenses and the status of funds?
H. What is the condition of equipment upon delivery and what is the nature of warranties?

meet their own learning objectives. The authors recognize that because of the outline's comprehensiveness, it may seem overwhelming to some. Thus you may wish to refer to textbooks in order to learn more about some of the areas included in the outline before proceeding with curriculum planning.

LEARNING ACTIVITIES

An important learning activity in computer education is the opportunity to become comfortable and familiar with computer systems. Students should have an opportunity for hands-on experience with a computer (micro, mainframe, or both). A vital part of computer education is reducing students' fears of the technology and improving their affective response to automation. It is important to remember that there is a constant interplay between computer concepts and applications. The instructor should always be cognizant of the need to reinforce knowledge of technical aspects of the computer when teaching applications. There are several means of providing interactive computer experiences: demonstration only, directed hands-on classroom exercises, and out-of-class assignments.

Demonstration only. There may be occasions when regular access to the computer is not possible and the instructor may need to use alternative methods to simulate interactive computer experiences. The instructor can demonstrate various software packages to students. This can be done using either a microcomputer or a terminal connected to a mainframe. It is also possible to connect a microcomputer to a large projection screen or television monitors so that more students can view the demonstration. Computers in a networking configuration can also be used. If educators do not have access to any computer systems, other audiovisual materials can be used to show the use of computers.

Directed classroom exercises. In some schools, students have computer lab exercises as part of their classroom time (Holzemer et al., 1984). They work individually or in pairs on directed activities supervised by the instructor. These activities may include exercises for keyboarding, the operating system, word processing or editing, and so forth (Skiba, 1985). Hands-on activities in the classroom offer many advantages. Initial interactive experiences for students are more likely to be positive ones, and the frustration level is likely to be kept to a minimum when the faculty member is available for consultation and guidance. In addition, computer concepts can be reinforced at this time so that students will better understand how the computer operates.

Out-of-class assignments. In addition to classroom activities, the students, either individually or in groups, may be assigned to complete a word processing, database management, or spreadsheet assignment as part of their coursework (Lange & Marks, 1986). This requires them to work without the instructor's on-site support while developing additional skill with the computer.

The type and extent of interactive computer experiences will depend on several factors: philosophy of the instructors, accessibility and availability of both hardware and software, specific learning objectives, faculty expertise, and the development of interactive exercises. In particular, the detailed assessment of resources described later in this chapter may alter the decisions about interactive computer experiences. Refer to the following resources for ideas for the development of interactive computer experiences: Grobe, 1984; Holzemer et al., 1984; Lange and Marks, 1986; Skiba, 1985; Theile, 1984.

After learning activities are selected, it is important to review the preselected point on the continuum, the objectives, the content, and the learning activities to ensure that they are mutually congruent. Since curriculum planning is a dynamic process with many feedback loops, verification of the internal consistency of the curriculum must be ongoing. If, at any point, there is lack of congruence among the major components of the curriculum, modifications will have to be made.

PLACEMENT IN THE CURRICULUM

After congruence among the various elements of the curriculum has been verified, it is time to analyze the placement of the content within the nursing curriculum. To facilitate the decision about where content on computers will be placed, two issues must be addressed: **time** and **timing**. Time refers to the number of class hours and timing refers to where in the curriculum the content is to be offered.

Time. The determination of how many class hours are needed to meet the learning objectives will be influenced by the breadth and depth of the course and whether the course is to be required or elective. This may require a careful evaluation of the curriculum, and the faculty may have to make compromises to place the content in an already tight curriculum.

Timing. Whether the computer course is to be elective or required, it is essential for the faculty to determine when the computer content will be taught. It is necessary for faculty to decide on the best fit of the content with all of the students' learning experiences. For example, it seems inappropriate to teach students about computer applications in nursing during the freshman and sophomore years if the students have not yet had exposure to nursing content. Basic computer concepts, though, could be taught during the freshman and sophomore years and the nursing applications could be introduced during the senior year. This example highlights a critical point: computer concepts can be taught separately from nursing applications. In some instances, students may take an introductory course in computer science as part of their liberal arts requirement before entering the nursing major.

Another necessary decision is whether the content will be taught as a separate course or will be integrated within existing courses. There are several advantages and disadvantages to each of these choices, and it is important for the faculty to agree on the best approach for their particular curriculum. To help make the decision, the following considerations should be kept in mind:

- Should basic computer concepts be taught separately from nursing applications?

- Should computer applications in nursing be taught as a separate course or integrated within existing courses, such as research or administration?

- Are faculty members available to teach the various options?

- Is there time within the nursing major to cover all topics necessary?

- How will the nursing emphasis be affected if the course is taught by non-nurses?

- If computer content is included in several different courses, is there continuity across that content?

A review of the nursing literature on computer education reveals several articles about this topic, but few research studies are available to support the different educational approaches and curricula espoused in the literature. Several articles describe an individual school's or hospital's approach to educating nurses about computers (see Appendix A). According to Heller et al. (1985), three basic approaches have been used to introduce computer content into the nursing curriculum: to offer an elective course, to require a general course on computers that is offered to all students in the college, and to integrate the computer content into existing nursing courses. Individual schools will have to decide whether one of these approaches or something different is appropriate for their particular setting.

DETAILED ASSESSMENT OF RESOURCES

As a next step it is crucial to conduct a detailed assessment of resources. This is a continuation of the preliminary assessment, but it is a more formal procedure that requires the collection of necessary data to facilitate decision making.

The detailed assessment of resources, both faculty as well as computer, can be carried out simultaneously with determination of what computer content is to be covered. It is also possible that some previous decisions will be revised based on the detailed analysis. As noted in Felton's (1984) chart, numerous questions can be included in the detailed assessment. The last three sections of this checklist can serve as an excellent guide for data collection (Fig. 2–3).

Faculty Resources

As a first step, it is critical to determine if there are faculty members who are supportive of computer technology and have the knowledge and skills to implement the computer content. It is essential to assess the entire faculty's attitudes toward and acceptance of computers, their experiences with computers, and their knowledge level and skills in computers.

Faculty attitudes toward computers. It has been documented that faculty members' attitude or acceptance of computer technology can be a factor in the implementation of computers within the curriculum and the use of computer assisted instruction as a teaching tool (Murphy, 1984). An assessment of the faculty will provide useful information for possible faculty development workshops and for the ultimate determination of who will be responsible for teaching computer content. Several attitude tools can be adapted to meet individual schools' needs (Ball, Snelbecker, & Schechter, 1985; Chang, 1984; Delaney, 1987; Kacynski & Roy, 1984; Stronge & Brodt, 1985; Whiteside & James, 1985/1986). The assessment should include a determination of faculty members' attitudes toward computer technology, the use of computers in nursing, and integration of computer concepts and computer applications in the curriculum.

Faculty experience with computers. A second assessment category is the type and amount of experience that the faculty has with computer technology. Some faculty members have only had exposure to computers in their own graduate work— data analysis using statistical software or exposure to word processing. Others have been exposed to computer technology in a clinical setting— experience with a hospital information system. The collection of these data will facilitate decision making in two distinct areas: determining which faculty members can teach what content as well as what type of faculty development is needed before beginning a course offering for students. Faculty development is man-

Figure 2-3. Felton's checklist for computer planning (Part II).

IV. Operation and implementation:

A. What other computing equipment on campus will be compatible with the intended purchase?

B. How long, typically, will you have to wait to get the equipment repaired—are components readily available?

C. Who will be able to hook it up to other equipment, as necessary?

D. Where will the item be located?

E. Will this location encourage its proper and most effective use?

F. Is this place secure?

G. Will you need some way of locking it in place? (Who will design the locking device and install it?)

H. Will the equipment be in view of some responsible person at all times?

I. Where will any associated supplies be kept—discs, manuals, extra connecting cables, printer paper, etc.?

J. Will it be necessary to check out supplies or equipment?

K. Who will accept this responsibility?

V. Software:

A. Is software available to support the intended use of the equipment?

B. What is the initial cost of the software?

C. Who will pay for additional software or updates?

D. Should upgrading of software be needed, who will do it and who will pay for it?

E. What possibilities exist for authorizing of software in the department? What help is available for those individuals?

Figure 2-3. *(continued)*

VI. **Miscellaneous problems:**

  A. Will this system in particular require much repair?

  B. Who is qualified to repair it?

  C. Are there any repair manuals on campus specific to this equipment?

  D. Who will replace it if it is lost or damaged?

  E. Who will do any required reprogramming to make the software compatible with this particular brand or with your department's particular needs?

  F. Will the computer need to be mobile? (Is it small and rugged enough to be moved around on an ordinary cart?)

  G. Will this require the installation of connecting lines or a telephone?

  H. What else must be purchased or created to make this acquisition fully operational?

datory for the successful integration of computers within the nursing curriculum. Therefore a thorough needs assessment of faculty will be beneficial to the entire change process.

An example of a needs assessment tool for faculty experiences with computers is provided in Appendix C. This tool includes just a few of the applications that faculty members can be asked about. Numerous surveys and articles mention types of applications to be included in a faculty needs assessment (Parks, Damrosch, Heller, & Romano, 1986; Ronald, 1983).

The needs assessment tool should include a section on the type of experience as well as the extent or frequency of that experience. It is also important to determine how recently the experiences took place. Because changes in computer technology occur at a rapid pace, it is crucial to determine if faculty members need updates in technology.

Faculty knowledge and skill. It is equally important to assess the faculty's level of knowledge and skills relevant to each of the content areas in Chapter 3. It is crucial for the faculty to feel comfortable with many of the chosen topics, as faculty members do not like to feel that students know more than they do. The assessment tool should determine the faculty's knowledge and skills with respect to:

1. Computer components and operations
2. Algorithmic design and flowcharting
3. Applications to clinical practice, administration, education, and research
4. Professional issues

Computer Resources

Computer resources, both hardware and software, must be evaluated for availability and accessibility to both faculty and students. The results of this analysis will help determine the extent and nature of computer interactive experiences possible for nursing students.

Availability. The key question is: Are there computer resources available for educational purposes? For example, the school of nursing may own five microcomputers but all may be used for administrative purposes; thus they are not available for student or classroom use. It is equally important to assess availability of resources across several locations: within the school of nursing, within the academic institution, in the community (libraries, computer societies, adult education classes), and in health care institutions. In addition to availability, the following information should be obtained: contact person, number of terminals and systems; manufacturer, type, memory capacity, printers, and type of video display terminal. Appendix D illustrates the types of information that can be collected. You may want to incorporate information about hardware availability at this time.

You should also simultaneously collect information about software availability. Again, it is important to remember that "available" means available for educational purposes. It is also essential to collect information about generic software (word processing, spreadsheets, and database management software that can be adapted for nursing use). As you gather information about available software, you must collect information about the hardware required to operate the software. Hardware requirements include such items as computer system, memory, printer, monitor, other peripherals, and operating system requirements.

Below is an example of a format that might be used to collect data about software availability and requirements.

Software	Location	Purpose	Hardware Requirements
Drug Calculations	Nursing	CAI-Drill	IBM-PC (256K), color monitor, printer not necessary, MS-DOS

It would also be to your advantage to note how this software could be applied to nursing. One could begin to investigate the fit between the type of software available and the nursing content area.

Accessibility. In addition to ascertaining availability, it is essential to determine accessibility. This includes answering questions about whether hardware and software are accessible to nursing students and faculty. If resources are accessible, how often and during what times? Are there any policies governing accessibility? Who is responsible for policies, scheduling time, or access? Access must also be examined in terms of public access (students can use the equipment individually), limited or reserved access (students must sign up in advance for access to the computer system), and classroom access (faculty members can reserve the use of a classroom laboratory for educational purposes).

Fees and support services. Once access has been determined, one must inquire about fees for the use of the computer systems and the support services that are available. The fees associated with the use of computer resources vary across institutions. Some colleges provide computer access to all students without additional charges. In other instances, students are charged a laboratory fee if the course requires the use of computer systems. Costs of access will greatly influence the extent and nature of interactive computer experiences chosen for students. In some cases, costs associated with use of computer resources outside of the school of nursing are extremely prohibitive and the school may consider the purchase of its own computer resources.

The other area of concern involves support services. When assessing resources, one should determine if the following support services are available and if there are any costs associated with the services:

- Technical assistance (help for faculty and students with the use of hardware and software). If such assistance is available, how much, how often, when and where, and to whom?

- Educational offerings (tutorial or practice sessions for both faculty and students on existing computer equipment or introduction to new equipment). Again, if available, how often, how much, when and where, and to whom?

- Maintenance assistance (services for the maintenance of both hardware and software resources). For example, you have reserved the computer lab for your class and three printers do not work. Whom do you call, what are the fees, and so forth.

IMPLEMENTATION

After deciding when, where, and how the content and learning activities will be integrated into the curriculum, the faculty will make plans for implementation. At this time, the faculty will decide what specific resources (textbooks, outside readings, audiovisual materials, and computer software) are to be used. It may be necessary to consult with the librarian to request the addition of relevant journals, conference proceedings, and books to the library's collection. A staged purchase plan may be needed, since computer publications are expensive and most nursing libraries have limited, if any, holdings in this area. Audiovisual materials and computer software will also have to be purchased.

Arrangements for use of computer facilities will have to be made well in advance. In most settings, computer availability for instructional use is limited and scheduled far in advance. It may be necessary to schedule class time based on the availability of the computer. Specific nursing-related computer exercises will have to be found. Textbooks, journals, colleagues, and meetings are the best resources for these. However, good nursing exercises are few and far between, and it may be necessary to develop your own.

In certain instances, schools of nursing may decide that it is to their advantage to establish a computer lab specifically for their students (Bitter, 1985; Stronge, Bell, & Keane, 1986). Availability, access, and cost factors may hinder the use of external facilities; therefore, a computer laboratory within the school may be the best alternative. Computer labs in a school of nursing can take several forms (Abraham & Fitzgerald, 1985; Bergin, 1985; Stronge et al., 1986). One form is a reserved terminal or microcomputer room: the placement of a limited number of microcomputers or terminals connected to the mainframe in a room whose access is limited to faculty and students of the school of nursing. The university or school provides the equipment but does not provide any support services, such as teaching assistants or technical services.

Another form, the computer-dedicated classroom, is set up to provide theoretical presentations that can be interspersed with interactive computer experiences for students. Use of this type of facility assumes that a sufficient number of terminals or micro-computers are available to accommodate the students in the classes. The computer-dedicated classroom may also include a local area network or a projection screen connected to the computer used by the faculty. The number of terminals or micro-computers considered sufficient depends on the goals of the computer classroom and the number of students to be serviced by the facility. Bergin (1985) has suggested that a good ratio of students to terminals is 3:1. Hales (1984) has offered the following formula for determining the number of computer systems necessary for a minimal installation.

First, multiply the number of students you wish to serve by the number of hours per week each student will be using the computer:

$$\text{Students} \times \text{Hours per week} = \text{Usage}$$

Second, calculate availability by multiplying the number of hours per week that the computers will be available by .75, since it is unrealistic to assume 100 percent availability:

$$\text{Hours per week} \times .75 = \text{Availability}$$

Third, divide Usage by Availability to determine the number of computer systems needed:

$$\frac{\text{Usage}}{\text{Availability}} = \text{Number of computer systems}$$

For example, if you have 50 students, each of whom will use the computer 3 hours per week, and the computer lab will be open 40 hours per week, you would calculate the number of computers needed as follows:

$$\text{Usage} = \frac{50 \times 3}{40 \times .75} = \frac{150}{30} = 5 \text{ computers}$$

A third alternative is to establish a computer resource learning lab that expands the previous alternatives by incorporating support services to assist faculty and student users. This lab can be operated in both a classroom mode and as an open resource for faculty and students. The computer resource lab also incorporates the notion of a library of resources, such as software and other instructional materials. The establishment of this type of facility will depend upon budget, resources, and staffing availability.

Given differences across academic institutions, it is important for each school to decide which alternative is the most appropriate for meeting the learning needs of its students. No matter which alternative is chosen, the following guidelines will be useful in planning a computer facility within the school of nursing (Bergin, 1985; Peters & Eddin, 1981).

Step 1. Conduct a needs assessment to determine the specific needs of courses using the lab, the number of students, and the type of computer support required.

Step 2. Assess current resources, including faculty, computer hardware and software, staffing, space, and budget considerations.

Step 3. Develop a strategic plan that includes the goals of the lab and an implementation plan.

Step 4. Determine available support. The creation of a computer lab requires considerable time and resources, both in people and dollars. Support must be solicited from administration and faculty to create this facility. Since many schools have limited budgets, external sources may have to be tapped for the funding of the facility. It is also advised that schools seek consultation at this phase to facilitate the development of the lab. Consultation will be beneficial in terms of design, funding sources, selection of hardware and software, policies, and structural design of the lab.

Step 5. Select software, hardware, and other resources needed to furnish the lab (e.g., computer tables).

Step 6. Determine the structural design of the lab. It is important to take ergonomic factors into consideration when designing the computer lab. Electricity, lighting, antistatic carpeting, ventilation, and furnishing requirements are just a few of the considerations. Modification of an existing environment may be required.

Step 7. Determine staffing and budgetary considerations.

Step 8. Develop an implementation plan (install equipment; train staff, and write policies for scheduling, computer usage, access, purchasing, and security).

Step 9. Implement, plan, and manage resources, including maintenance policies, technical support and assistance, operating budget considerations, and future development plans.

Step 10. Evaluate computer lab in terms of effectiveness and efficiency. Detailed statistics should be kept about amount and type of usage, number of students, repairs, and so forth.

EVALUATION

Evaluation of the computer aspects of the curriculum will need to be done every semester. Because of the rapidly changing nature of the computer field, both the cognitive and interactive components of computer content will differ from year to year and often from semester to semester. Factors that affect this and that should be considered in the evaluation and subsequent revisions include changes in program goals, incoming student behaviors, computer technology, health care applications (local and national), employers' expectations of new graduates, availability and accessibility of computer resources for teaching, and availability of new textbooks, journals, and computer software.

SUMMARY

The preceding chapters have described flexible guidelines for educators to use in integrating computer concepts into the curriculum. Initially a computer education framework based on specific assumptions was described. This was followed by explanations and illustrations to clarify the framework. Next, the elements of the curriculum decision making process were presented in a flowchart format. This was followed by a discussion of the specific steps delineated in the diagram.

In the chapter that follows, a detailed outline of content will be presented. The authors have included a separate chapter on content because this is the area in which nursing educators have asked for the most assistance.

3

Content Guidelines

Chapter 3 contains a generic topical outline of computer content areas. These areas were selected primarily with the proficient user in the middle of the computer education continuum in mind. Although every attempt has been made to make the outline comprehensive, it is not meant to be an exhaustive list of all content relevant for nurses; neither is it meant to imply that each element in it must be included in the curriculum for a proficient user. The sample learning activities extend over the entire continuum and show different levels of sophistication within the content areas.

The outline is intended to be modified by faculty members to meet their own learning objectives. At the present time there is no established curriculum for nurses, at any level of expertise. While some readers might prefer a more prescriptive approach to content, the authors do not believe that this is possible. The research data available upon which to base computer competencies for nurses is limited. In addition, curriculum factors identified in the preceding chapter, particularly resources, differ significantly from institution to institution. This affects the content selected and the depth in which it can be offered.

When reviewing this chapter, you may find it useful to refer to textbooks to gain a clearer understanding of some of the areas included. This will also help you become familiar with the breadth and depth of content in the different books that are available.

CONTENT OUTLINE

I. **Historical Perspectives**

    A. *Computers*

        1. Eniac (electronic numerical integrator and calculator)
        2. Transistors
        3. Integrated circuits
        4. Microprocessors
        5. Knowledge information processing systems

    B. *Computer applications to nursing and health care*

        1. Financial applications
        2. Ancillary services
        3. Physiological monitoring
        4. Information systems
            a. Communication
            b. Clinical data
        5. Decision support

    C. *Acceptance of computerization*

        1. Attitudes of nurses
        2. Relationship to history of nursing
        3. Humanistic vs. technological orientation

II. **The Computer**

    A. *Unique characteristics of the computer*

        1. Memory
        2. Speed
        3. Repetitiveness
        4. Automaticity
        5. Accuracy

      6. Decision making

B. Basic operations of the computer

      1. Information storage and retrieval

      2. Calculation

      3. Logical operations

C. Information processing

      1. Data vs. information

      2. Processing cycle

      3. Information processing in nursing

D. Hardware components

      1. Input devices

        a. Function

        b. Types

      2. Output devices

        a. Function

        b. Types

      3. Central processing unit

        a. Function

        b. Components

          (1) Control unit

          (2) Arithmetic/logic unit

      4. Internal memory

        a. Function

        b. Characteristics

        c. Types

          (1) ROM

          (2) RAM

      5. External memory (auxiliary storage)

        a. Function

        b. Characteristics

        c. Types

          (1) Magnetic disks

          (2) Magnetic tapes

E. Hardware configuration

      1. Types

        a. Analog

        b. Digital

2. Sizes
   a. Mainframe computer
   b. Minicomputer
   c. Microcomputer

F. Data representation in the computer

1. Binary
   a. Concept
   b. Numbering system
2. Bits and bytes
3. Binary coded systems
   a. Types (ASCII, EBCDIC)
   b. Functions
   c. Internal representation of data
      (1) Data cycle: keyboard stroke to output

G. Software development

1. Function of software
2. Programming languages
   a. Levels
      (1) Machine
      (2) Assembly
      (3) Higher level
   b. Interpreted vs. compiled languages
3. Programming process
   a. Problem
   b. Algorithm
   c. Flowchart
   d. Code
   e. Debugging
   f. Documenting
4. Programming skills
   a. Structured programming
   b. Applications languages
   c. Boolean logic

H. System configuration

1. Types
   a. Stand-alone
   b. Networks
   c. Distributed
2. Advantages and disadvantages

III. Systems Analysis and Design

A. *Stages*

1. Planning
2. Analysis
3. Design
4. Development
5. Implementation
6. Evaluation

B. *Roles*

1. User
2. Content expert
3. Information specialist
4. Programmer

SAMPLE LEARNING ACTIVITIES FOR SECTIONS
II AND III

1. Tour of computer facilities
2. Demonstration of computer parts and functions
3. Videotape: "Computer Concepts for Health Care Professionals," available from Ozz Associates, Austin, Texas
4. Hands-on exercises with micro and/or mainframe computer
   a. Keyboarding
   b. Operating system exercises
   c. Wordprocessing/editing
   d. Running computer programs, such as "The Glass Computer," a CAI program available from the Minnesota Educational Computer Consortium, other CAI packages, and various games
   e. Writing a simple program
5. Development of algorithms and flowcharts
   a. General
   b. Nursing

IV. Application of Computers to Nursing

A. Clinical applications

1. Physiological monitoring
   a. Surveillance
   b. Diagnosis
   c. Treatment
2. Documentation of the nursing process
   a. Nursing assessment
   b. Nursing care plans
   c. Recording nursing observations, activities, and decisions
   d. Evaluation of nursing care
3. Health care information systems
   a. Types of information
      (1) Health care
      (2) Nursing
         (a) Patient care
         (b) Unit management
         (c) Administration
   b. Hospital information systems
      (1) Classification of hospital information systems
      (2) Conceptual basis of systems
      (3) Prototype systems
         (a) El Camino Hospital
         (b) National Institutes of Health
         (c) PROMIS system
   c. Ambulatory health care systems
      (1) Costar
      (2) Automated Multiphasic Health Testing
      (3) Automated histories
   d. Community health information systems
      (1) Remote patient monitoring
      (2) Omaha Visiting Nurse Association
4. Decision support
   a. Continuum: decision assisting to decision making
   b. Clinical databases
      (1) Aggregated clinical experience
      (2) Nursing database
         (a) Current status

        (b) Problems
        (c) Potential
    c. Artificial intelligence— expert systems
       (1) Definition
       (2) Medical systems
          (a) Mycin
          (b) Internist
          (c) Help
       (3) Nursing system
          (a) Commes

5. Impact of clinical applications
    a. Patient
    b. Nurse
    c. Nursing profession
    d. Health care

SAMPLE LEARNING ACTIVITIES FOR SECTION IVA

1. Field trip to local health care agency with a computer
2. Group exercise to identify standardized nursing content for a specific nursing care problem
3. Hands-on computer experience with clinical applications
    a. Demonstration packages from vendors
    b. Local health care agencies with computerized information systems

B. Administrative applications

1. Management information systems
    a. Definition
    b. Function
    c. Stand-alone vs. integrated systems
2. Administrative components
    a. Scheduling
    b. Staffing
        (1) Patient acuity
        (2) Staff profile
    c. Quality assurance
    d. Administrative reports
    e. Budgeting and forecasting/modeling
    f. Decision-support systems for management
    g. Record keeping and database management
    h. Resource management

SAMPLE LEARNING ACTIVITIES FOR SECTION IVB

1. Hands-on activities (Skiba, 1985; Lange & Marks, 1986)
   a. Database management system (patient records, personnel records)
   b. Spread sheet (budgeting)
   c. Project management packages
   d. Graphics

C. *Educational applications*

1. Uses in education
   a. Teaching with computers
   b. Testing
   c. Managing instruction
2. Definition of terms and acronyms
   a. CAI: Computer-assisted instruction
   b. CMI: Computer-managed instruction
   c. CAL: Computer-assisted learning
   d. CBL: Computer-based learning
3. Teaching with computers (CAI)
   a. Effectiveness of CAI
   b. Types of CAI
      (1) Drill and practice
      (2) Tutorial
      (3) Gaming
      (4) Simulation
      (5) Problem solving
      (6) Interactive video
   c. Benefits of CAI
   d. Uses of CAI
      (1) Nursing education
      (2) Inservice education
      (3) Continuing education
      (4) Patient education
   e. CAI development
      (1) Instructional design
      (2) Authoring languages
      (3) Authoring systems
   f. Evaluation of software
4. Testing
   a. Test generation

   b. Item analysis
   c. Automated testing
5. Managing instruction: computer-managed instruction
   a. Monitor student progress
   b. Diagnose learning needs
   c. Prescribe learning materials
6. Implementation
   a. Curriculum planning
   b. Software selection
   c. Faculty role

SAMPLE LEARNING ACTIVITIES FOR SECTION IVC
1. Hands-on computer experience
   a. CAI
   b. Test development programs
   c. Authoring systems
2. CAI evaluation exercise
3. CAI development exercise
(Some of the above are available from publishing companies on demonstration disks)

D. *Research applications*
1. Information retrieval
   a. Bibliographic databases
   b. Patient databases
2. Data collection
3. Data analysis
4. Graphics
5. Report writing

SAMPLE LEARNING ACTIVITIES FOR SECTION IVD
1. On-line library search
2. Extraction of data from a research file
3. Statistical analysis using SPSS, SAS, EPISTAT
4. Graphics generation

E. *Communications*
1. Timesharing
2. Distributed systems
3. Networking: local area networks (LAN)

    4. Telecommunications
      a. Hardware
      b. Software
      c. Services
        (1) Patient databanks
        (2) Information retrieval systems
        (3) Electronic mail
        (4) Teleconferencing
        (5) Bulletin boards

SAMPLE LEARNING ACTIVITIES FOR SECTION IVE

1. Bibliographic search, e.g. Grateful Med (available from National Library of Medicine for a nominal fee)
2. Access information services if available, e.g. COMPUSERVE

V. Role of the Nurse

A. Selection and development of a system

1. Nursing membership on hospital computer committee
2. Analysis of nursing needs
3. Cost/benefit analysis of alternative systems
4. Evaluation of vendor's response to a request for proposal (RFP) from a nursing perspective
5. Adaptation of system to meet nursing's needs

B. Planning for implementation

C. Preparation of staff to work with the system

D. Ongoing evaluation of the system

E. Ongoing development of the system

SAMPLE LEARNING ACTIVITIES FOR SECTION V

1. Investigate membership and functions of local health care agencies' computer committees
2. Identify selected nursing information requirements for an automated information system
3. Role play the selection of a system from a vendor
4. Do a needs assessment for a nursing information system

   5. Write a nursing section for an RFP

VI. Professional Issues Related to the Use of Computers in Health Care

A. *Privacy, confidentiality, and security*

B. *Legal issues*

C. *Impact of computers on individuals, organizations, and society*

D. *Future professional roles*

SAMPLE LEARNING ACTIVITIES FOR SECTION VI

   1. Case studies of legal cases or ethical dilemmas
   2. Role panel of nurses working in the development and implementation of computerized systems

References

Abraham, I., & Fitzpatrick, J. (1985). Research environments in nursing: Rationale and requirements for computing. In M. Ackerman (Ed.); *Proceedings of the Ninth Annual Symposium on Computer Applications in Medical Care* (pp. 814–818). Los Angeles: IEEE Computer Society Press.

Ball, M., Snelbecker, G., & Schechter, S. (1985). Nurses' perceptions concerning computer use before and after a computer literacy lecture. *Computers in Nursing, 3*(1), 23–31.

Bergin, T. (1985). Establishing a computer science laboratory to support the teaching of the social sciences. *Social Science Microcomputer Review, 3*(1), 14–27.

Bitter, G. (1985). Computer labs—Fads? *Electronic Education, 4*(7), 17, 35.

Chang, B. (1984) Adoption of innovations: Nursing and computer use. *Computers in Nursing, 2*(6), 229–235.

Delaney, C. (1987). Administrator and faculty acceptance of the computer as a technological innovation in baccalaureate nursing programs in independent colleges in the Midwest (Abstract). *Pro-*

ceedings of the Fifth Annual Research in Nursing Education Conference (p. 48). New York: National League for Nursing.

Felton, B. (1984). Planning and implementing computer learning in a department of nursing. *Nursing & Health Care, 5*(10), 549–553.

Felton, G., & Brown, B. (1985). Application of computer technology in two colleges of nursing. *Journal of Nursing Education, 24*(1), 5–9.

Gothler, A. (1985). Nursing education update: Computer technology. *Nursing & Health Care, 6*(9), 509–510.

Grobe, S. (1984). Conquering computer cowardice. *Journal of Nursing Education, 23*(6), 232–239.

Hales, G., Tarp, J., & Smith, R. (1984). *Hardware Evaluation Checklist— Version 2.0.* Boston, MA: Boston University School of Nursing, Computer Applications in Nursing Institute.

Heller, B., Romano, C., Damrosch, S., & Parks, P. (1985). Computer applications in nursing: Implications for the curriculum. *Computers in Nursing, 3*(1), 14–21.

Holzemer, W. L., Slichter, M. J., Slaughter, R. E., Stotts, N. A., Chambers, D. B., & Scheetz, S. (1984). Development of a computer resource facility. *Nursing & Health Care, 5*(10), 545–547.

Johnson, B. (1984). Improving decision making in the dean's office. In G. Cohen (Ed.), *Proceedings of the Eighth Annual Symposium on Computer Applications in Medical Care* (pp. 610–613). Los Angeles: IEEE Computer Society Press.

Kacynski, K., & Roy, K. (1984) An analysis of graduate students' innovation-decision process. In G. Cohen (Ed.), *Proceedings of the Eighth Annual Symposium of Computer Applications in Medical Care* (pp. 605–609). Los Angeles: IEEE Computer Society Press.

Lange, L., & Mark, B. (1986). Teaching computer use in a graduate program in nursing administration. In R. Salamon, B. Blum, & M. Jorgensen (Eds.), *Proceedings of the Fifth Conference on Medical Informatics (MEDINFO 86)* (pp. 917–919). Amsterdam, The Netherlands: North-Holland Publishers.

Masland, A. (1984). Encouraging innovative academic computing. *Educational Record, 65*(4), 36–41.

Murphy, M. (1984). Computer-based education in nursing: Factors influencing its utilization. *Computers in Nursing*, 2(6), 218–223.

Parks, P., Damrosch, S., Heller, B., & Romano, C. (1986). Comparison of nursing faculty and student definitions of computer learning needs. In R. Salamon, B. Blum, & M. Jorgensen (Eds.), *Proceedings of the Fifth Conference on Medical Informatics (MEDINFO 86)* (pp. 950–954). Amsterdam, The Netherlands: North-Holland Publishers.

Peters, G., & Eddin, J. (1981). *A planning guide to successful computer instruction.* Champaign, IL: Electronic Courseware Systems.

Ronald, J. (1983). Learning needs and attitudes of nursing educators with respect to computers. In R. Dayhoff (Ed.), *Proceedings of the Seventh Annual Symposium of Computer Applications in Medical Care* (pp. 523–526). Los Angeles: IEEE Computer Society Press.

Skiba, D. (1985). Interactive computer experiences: The missing ingredient. *Nursing Clinics of North America*, 20(3), 577–584.

Stronge, J., Bell, S., & Keane, D. (1986). School computers— Success often depends on location. *Electronic Education*, 5(7), 12–13, 22.

Stronge, J., & Brodt, A. (1985). Assessment of nurses' attitudes toward computerization. *Computers in Nursing*, 3(4), 154–158.

Theile, J., & Baldwin, J. (1984). A simulated practice environment: Computerville Regional Hospital. *Computers in Nursing*, 3(3), 113–116.

Torres, G., & Stanton, M. (1982). *Curriculum process in nursing.* Englewood Cliffs, NJ: Prentice-Hall.

Vakos, H. N. (1986). Ten steps to putting together a comprehensive plan for computer education. *T.H.E. Journal*, 13(6), 56–59.

Walker, M. (1986). Nursing education: Challenges of the computerized environment. *Computers in Nursing*, 4(4), 166–171.

Whiteside, C., & James, R. (1985/1986). Utilizing teachers' concerns to improve microcomputer implementation. *Computers in the Schools*, 2(4), 29–41.

APPENDIX A

Resources on Computer Literacy

Anderson, J., Gremy, F., & Pages, J. C. (1974). *Education in Informatics of Health Professionals.* New York: American Elsevier Co.

Arnold, J. M., & Bauer, C. A. (1985). Computer literacy needs of nurse educators and nurse managers. In M. Ackerman (Ed.), *Proceedings of the Ninth Annual Symposium on Computer Applications in Medical Care* (pp. 829–834). Los Angeles: IEEE Computer Society Press.

Barnett, G. O., Piggins, J., Moore, G., Foster, E., Kozaczka, J., & Scott, J. (1986). Information technology in a new curriculum—An experiment in medical education. In R. Salamon, B. Blum, & M. Jorgensen (Eds.), *Proceedings of the Fifth Conference on Medical Informatics (MEDINFO 86)* (pp. 883–886). Amsterdam, The Netherlands: North-Holland Publishers.

Bergin, T. J. (1985). Establishing a computer science laboratory to support the teaching of the social sciences. *Social Science Microcomputer Review, 3*(1), 14–27.

Blum, B. I. (1984). Understanding computer basics. *MD Computing, 1*(1), 59–65.

Bowman, R. F. (1985). Computer literacy: A strategy for cultivating consensus. *T.H.E. Journal, 13*, 60–62.

Brose, C. (1984). Computer technology in nursing: Revolution or renaissance. *Nursing & Health Care, 5*(10), 531–534.

Cheng, T., & Stevens, D. J. (1985). Prioritizing computer literacy topics. *Computers & Education, 9*(1), 9–13.

Earp, J. (1985). Nursing education—The computer obligation (Editorial). *Computers in Nursing, 3*(5), 196, 232.

Feeg, V. (1984). The computer education challenge to nursing education: What? when? how? and why? *Computers in Nursing, 2*(3), 88–91.

Felton, B. (1984). Planning and implementing computer learning in a department of nursing. *Nursing & Health Care, 5*(10), 549–553.

Felton, G., & Brown, B. J. (1985). Application of computer technology in two colleges of nursing. *Journal of Nursing Education, 24*(1), 5–9.

Gothler, A. (1985). Nursing education update: Computer technology. *Nursing & Health Care, 6*(9), 509–510.

Grobe, S. (1984). Conquering computer cowardice. *Journal of Nursing Education, 23*(6), 232–238.

Hales, G. (1986). Nursing information systems: The key to the future (Editorial). *Computers in Nursing, 4*(3), 102–136.

Hannah, K. J. (1983). The placement of medical informatics in a baccalaureate nursing curriculum. In J. C. Pages, A. H. Levy, & J. Anderson (Eds.), *Meeting the Challenge: Informatics and Medical Education.* New York: Elsevier Science Publishing.

Hardin, R. C., & Skiba, D. J. (1982). A comparative analysis of computer literacy education for nurses. In B. Blum (Ed.), *Proceedings of the Sixth Annual Symposium on Computer Applications in Medical Care* (pp. 525–530). Los Angeles: IEEE Computer Society Press.

Heller, B., Romano, C., Damrosch, S., & Parks, P. (1985). Computer applications in nursing: Implications for the curriculum. *Computers in Nursing, 3*(1), 14–25.

Holzemer, W., Slichter, M. J., Slaughter, R. E., Stotts, N. A.,

Chambers, D. B., & Scheetz, S. (1984). Development of a computer resources facility. *Nursing & Health Care*, *5*(10), 545–547.

Jackson, W., Clements, D., & Jones, L. (1984–85). Computer awareness and use at a research university. *Journal of Educational Technology Systems*, *13*(1), 47–57.

Kellogg, B., & Garcia, S. (1985). Introducing nursing students to computers. *Computers in Nursing*, *3*(3), 128–132.

Kirk, L., Abraham, I., Jane, L., & Fitzpatrick, J. (1986). Comprehensive computerization of a school of nursing: Planning aspects and system description. In R. Salamon, B. Blum, & M. Jorgensen (Eds.), *Proceedings of the Fifth Conference on Medical Informatics (MEDINFO 86)* (pp. 972–974). Amsterdam, The Netherlands: North-Holland Publishers.

Koch, P. (1984). The missing ingredient in computer education: The affective domain. In G. Cohen (Ed.), *Proceedings of the Eighth Annual Symposium on Computer Applications in Medical Care* (pp. 676–678). Los Angeles: IEEE Computer Society Press.

Lange, L., & Mark, B. (1986). Teaching computer use in a graduate program in nursing administration. In R. Salamon, B. Blum, & M. Jorgensen (Eds.), *Proceedings of the Fifth Conference on Medical Informatics (MEDINFO 86)* (pp. 917–919). Amsterdam, The Netherlands: North-Holland Publishers.

Lenkway, P. (1986). Minimum student performance standards in computer literacy: Florida's new state law. *T.H.E. Journal*, *13*, 74–77.

Lockheed, M., & Mandinach, E. (1986). Trends in educational computing: Decreasing interest and the changing focus of instruction. *Educational Researcher*, *15*(5), 21–26.

Luehrman, A. (1980). Pre- and post-college computer education. In R. Taylor (Ed.), *The Computer in the School: Tutor, Tool, Tutee* (pp. 141–148). New York: Teachers College Press.

Martin, C. D., & Heller, R. S. (1982). Computer literacy for teachers. *Educational Leadership*, *39*, 45–49.

McAlister, N., & Cory, P. (1986). Teaching medical computing to medical students. In R. Salamon, B. Blum, & M. Jorgensen (Eds.), *Proceedings of the Fifth Conference on Medical Informatics (MEDINFO 86)* (pp. 960–965). Amsterdam, The Netherlands: North-Holland Publishers.

McKay, A., Speedie, S., & Kerr, R. (1986). Fostering computer literacy through the use of innovation opinion leaders. In R. Salamon, B. Blum, & M. Jorgensen (Eds.), *Proceedings of the Fifth Conference on Medical Informatics (MEDINFO 86)* (pp. 960–965). Amsterdam, The Netherlands: North-Holland Publishers.

Mikan, K. (1984). Computer integration: A challenge for nursing education. *Nursing Outlook, 32*(1), 6.

Neu, Emil C. (1985–86). A curriculum concept: The computer thread. *Journal of Educational Technology Systems, 14*(13), 187–192.

Newbern, V. (1985). Computer literacy in nursing education. *Nursing Clinics of North America, 20*(3), 549–536.

Parks, P., Damrosch, S., Heller, B., & Romano, C. (1986). Comparison of nursing faculty and student definitions of computer learning needs. In R. Salamon, B. Blum, & M. Jorgensen (Eds.), *Proceedings of the Fifth Conference on Medical Informatics (MEDINFO 86)* (pp. 950–954). Amsterdam, The Netherlands: North-Holland Publishers.

Romano, C. (1984). Computer technology and emerging roles: The challenge to nursing education. *Computers in Nursing, 2*(3), 80–84.

Ronald, J. (1981). Introducing nursing students to the use of computers in health care. In H. Hefferman (Ed.), *Proceedings of the Fifth Annual Symposium of Computer Applications in Medical Care* (pp. 771–775). Los Angeles: IEEE Computer Society Press.

Ronald, J. (1983a). Guidelines for computer literacy curriculums in a School of Nursing. *Journal of the New York State Nurses' Association, 14*(1), 12–18.

Ronald, J. (1983b). Learning needs and attitudes of nursing educators with respect to computers. In R. Dayhoff (Ed.), *Proceedings of the Seventh Annual Symposium on Computer Applications in Medical Care.* Los Angeles: IEEE Computer Society Press.

Ronald, J. (1985). Nursing education: The computer as catalyst. In K. Hannah, E. Guillemin, & D. Conklin (Eds.), *Nursing Use of Computers and Information Science* (pp. 523–529). Amsterdam: Elsevier Science Publishing.

Skiba, D. (1983). Computer literacy: The challenge of the 80's. *Journal of the New York State Nurses' Association, 14*(1), 6–11.

Skiba, D. (1984). The missing link. (Editorial). *Computers in Nursing, 2*(4), 117, 124.

Skiba, D. (1985). Interactive computer experiences: The missing ingredient. *Nursing Clinics of North America, 20*(3), 577–584.

Skiba, D., & Hardin, R. (1983). Development and implementation of a micro-based computer workshop series for nurses. In R. Dayhoff (Ed.), *Proceedings of the Seventh Annual Symposium of Computer Applications in Medical Care.* Los Angeles: IEEE Computer Society Press.

Sollet, P., & van Bremmel, J. (1986). Fourth-generation software for medical training programs. In R. Salamon, B. Blum, & M. Jorgensen (Eds.), *Proceedings of the Fifth Conference on Medical Informatics (MEDINFO 86)* (pp. 906–908). Amsterdam, The Netherlands: North-Holland Publishers.

Steibel, M., & Garhart, C. (1985). Beyond computer literacy. *T.H.E. Journal, 12*(6), 69–73.

Stronge, J., Bell, S., & Keane, D. (1986). School computers— Success often depends on location. *Electronic Education, 5*(7), 12–13, 22.

Vakos, H. N. (1986). Ten steps to putting together a comprehensive plan for computer education. *T.H.E. Journal, 13*(6), 56–59.

van Bemmel, J., Hasman, A., Sollet, P., & Veth, A. (1983). Training in medical informatics. *Computers and Biomedical Research, 16*, 414–432.

Walker, M. (1986). Nursing education: Challenges of the computerized environment. *Computers in Nursing, 4*(4), 166–171.

Zielstorff, R. (1976). Orienting personnel to automated systems. *Journal of Nursing Administration, 6*(2), 14–16.

Ziemer, M. (1984). Issues of computer literacy in nursing education. *Nursing & Health Care, 5*(10), 537–542.

APPENDIX B

Sample Resources on Computers in Nursing

BOOKS

Ball, M., & Hannah, K. (1984). *Using Computers in Nursing*. Philadelphia: J. B. Lippincott.

Billings, D. (1986). *Computer Assisted Instruction for Health Professionals*. Norwalk, CT: Appleton-Century-Crofts.

Bronzino, J. (1982). *Computer Applications for Patient Care*. Menlo Park, CA: Addison-Wesley.

Christensen, W., & Rupp, P. (1986). *The Nurse Manager's Guide to Computers*. Rockville, MD: Aspen.

Christensen, W., & Stearns, E. (1984). *Microcomputers in Health Care Management*. Rockville, MD: Aspen.

Dreyfus, H. L., & Dreyfus, S. E. (1986). *Mind Over Machine*. New York: Free Press.

Gallagher, S. (1983). *Inside the Personal Computer: A Pop-Up Guide*. New York: Abbeville Press.

Grobe, S. (1984). *Computer Primer and Resource Guide for Nurses*. Philadelphia: J. B. Lippincott.

Hannah, K., Guillemin, E., & Conklin, D. (Eds.). (1985). *Nursing Uses of Computers and Information Science.* New York: Elsevier.

Johnson, D. G., & Snapper, J. W. (1984). *Ethical Issues in the Use of Computers.* Monterey, CA: Wadsworth.

Pocklington, D., & Guttman, L. (1984). *Nursing Reference for Computer Literature.* Philadelphia: J. B. Lippincott.

Privacy Protection Study Commission. (1977). *Personal Privacy in an Information Society* (Stock No. 052-003-00395-3). Washington, DC: U.S. Government Printing Office.

Saba, V., & McCormick, K. A. (1986). *Essentials of Computers for Nurses.* Philadelphia: J. B. Lippincott.

Scholes, M., Bryant, Y., & Barber, B. (1983). *The Impact of Computers on Nursing: An International Review.* New York: Elsevier.

Sweeney, M. (1985). *The Nurse's Guide to Computers.* New York: Macmillan.

Walker, M., & Schwartz, C. (1984). *What Every Nurse Should Know About Computers.* Philadelphia: J. B. Lippincott.

Werley, H., & Grier, M. (1981). *Nursing Information Systems.* New York: Springer.

Westin, A. (1976). *Computers, Health Records, and Citizen Rights.* (National Bureau of Standards Monograph 157). Washington, DC: U.S. Government Printing Office.

Worthley, J. (1982). *Managing Computers in Health Care.* Ann Arbor, Michigan: Alpha Press.

Zielstorff, R. (Ed.). (1982). *Computers in Nursing.* Rockville, MD: Aspen.

COMPUTER-RELATED JOURNALS

Computers and Biomedical Research. Bimonthly international journal focusing on research done in the application of computers to biology and medicine. Sent to all members of AAMSI.

Computers in Biology and Medicine. Bimonthly international journal focusing on the application of the computer to the fields of bioscience and medicine. Includes a software survey form in each issue and periodically publishes software descriptions submitted by readers.

Computers in Healthcare. Monthly that focuses on computer applications in healthcare with special issues devoted to a particular type of system, such as nursing information systems, pharmacy, lab, ancillary.

Computers in Life Science Education. Monthly that focuses on the use of computer technology in the education of life science professionals such as physiologists, biologists, and nurses.

Computers and Medicine. Monthly that focuses on computer applications in medicine and health care. Includes announcements about meetings, new books, and other news relevant to the use of computers in medicine.

Computers in Nursing. Bimonthly that focuses on the uses of computers in nursing administration, education, practice, and research. In addition to articles, it contains important announcements about the latest happenings in nursing and computers as well as book and software reviews.

HealthCare Computing and Communications. Monthly that focuses on the use of computers by the health care system.

Journal of Clinical Computing. Bimonthly devoted to clinical applications in health care. Occasional special issues focused on specific clinical areas such as nursing.

Journal of Computer-Based Instruction. Quarterly devoted to the use of computers within educational environments. Special issues are devoted to such themes as health care, interactive video, and music instruction.

Journal of Educational Computing Research. Quarterly devoted to the presentation of research in the theory and applications of educational computing.

Journal of Educational Technology Systems. Quarterly devoted to the use of educational technology and its impact in the classroom.

Journal of Medical Systems. Quarterly devoted to the use of information systems within health care. Some issues focus on selected articles from conferences, such as the Symposium on Computer Applications in Medical Care and the Hawaii Information Systems Conference.

MD Computing. Bimonthly devoted to the use of computers in medical care. Contains information related to both the hospital and office practice, as well as basic information (tutorials) on computer concepts. Sent to all members of AAMSI.

Nurse Educator's MicroWorld. Bimonthly devoted to the use of microcomputers in nursing education. Practical suggestions for microcomputer use as well as news items and product information.

Social Science Microcomputer Review. Quarterly devoted to the use of computers in the social sciences. Numerous curriculum articles that have implications for nursing, as well as information about the National Collegiate Software Clearinghouse.

Software in Healthcare. Bimonthly devoted to software, systems, and communications in healthcare. Yearly directory of software companies and products.

T.H.E. (Technological Horizons in Education) Journal. Published ten times yearly and devoted to computer usage in education. Available free on a limited basis for educators.

PROFESSIONAL ORGANIZATIONS

ANA Council on Computer Applications in Nursing. The purpose of the council is to promote the use of computers in nursing practice and research as well as to serve as a resource on computer applications in nursing and provide professional development by sponsoring computer-related educational programs. The council publishes a bimonthly newsletter, *Input & Output.* ANA, Council Affiliation, ANA Fiscal Affairs, 2420 Pershing Road, Kansas City, MO 64108.

NLN National Forum on Computers in Health Care and Nursing. The purpose of the forum is to stimulate an awareness of the imperative to integrate technology into the thinking and actions of the nursing community and to develop systematic plans and programs to incorporate computer technology into the various aspects of nursing education and nursing service. National League for Nursing, 10 Columbus Circle, New York, NY 10019–1350.

American Association of Medical Systems and Informatics (AAMSI). AAMSI is a multidisciplinary organization focusing on computer applications in health care in three ways: developing scientific and educational programs; promoting the development and implementation of systems; and fostering medical computing and information technology through a multidisciplinary forum. There is a special interest group in nursing as part of AAMSI. AAMSI, Suite 700, 1101 Connecticut Ave., NW, Washington, DC 20036.

Association for the Development of Computer-Based Instructional Systems (ADCIS). ADCIS's goal is to promote the use of computer-based instruction at all levels of education. The organization has several special-interest groups that are of particular interest to health care professionals: Health Education; Interactive Video. ADCIS, Miller Hall 409, Western Washington University, Bellingham, WA 98225.

Special Interest Group, Computer Applications in Nursing (SIG-CIN). SIG-CIN is an informal organization whose primary goal is to promote networking among professional organizations and to foster the development of nurse-computer special interest groups in other organizations. SIG-CIN was established at the Fifth Annual Symposium on Computer Applications in Medical Care and has its annual meetings at the symposium. Diane J. Skiba, Treasurer, Graduate School of Nursing, University of Massachusetts at Worcester, 55 Lake Ave. North, Worcester, MA 01605–2397.

Association for Computing Machinery (ACM). The purposes of the ACM are to advance the sciences and art of information processing; to promote the free interchange of information about the sciences and art of information processing, and to develop and maintain the competence of information processing specialist. There is a special interest group in biomedical computing. Association for Computing Machinery, P.O. Box 9182, Church Street Station, New York, NY 10249.

APPENDIX C

Needs Assessment Tool for Faculty Experiences

Experiences	Mainframe	Micro
Research		
Statistical analysis		
Literature searches		
Database searches		
Telecommunications		
Graphics		
Instruction		
Use of CAI		
Developing CAI courseware		
Use of authoring software		
Test generation		
Test analysis		
Clinical practice/administration		
Hospital information systems		
Physiological monitoring equipment		
Nursing information systems		
Order entry systems		
Ancillary retrieval systems		
Patient care planning		
Staffing and scheduling		
Quality assurance		
Budgeting and financial management		

Experiences	Mainframe	Micro
Generic software usage		
Word processing		
Spreadsheets		
Database management systems		
File management system		
Programming		
Language known—e.g., BASIC, PASCAL		

APPENDIX D

Tool to Assess Computer Resources

Assessment of Mainframe and Minicomputer Resources

Location	Number of Terminals	Type		Printers		Contact Person
Library	25	10	VT100's	15		Dr. Byte
		15	DecWriters			
Computer Center	150	100	IBM3278's	50		Dr. Jones
		50	DecWriters	1	laser	

Assessment of Microcomputer Resources

Location	Manu-facturer	Num-ber	Mem-ory	Printers	Display Monitor	Contact Person
Nursing	MacIntosh	25	512K	18	monochrome	Dr. Smith
Library	IBM-PC	50	256K	25	1/2 color	Dr. Jones
					1/2 mono-chrome	

DATE DUE